Nursing & Health Survival Guide

Essential Clinical Skills

Susan Carlisle

Harlow, England • London • New York • Boston • San Francisco • Toronto • Sydney
Auckland • Singapore • Hong Kong • Tokyo • Seoul • Taipei • New Delhi
Cape Town • São Paulo • Mexico City • Madrid • Amsterdam • Munich • Paris • Milan

Pearson Education Limited
Edinburgh Gate
Harlow
Essex CM20 2JE
England

and Associated Companies throughout the world

Visit us on the World Wide Web at:
www.pearson.com/uk

First published 2012

ISBN 978-0-273-76881-4

British Library Cataloguing-in-Publication Data
A catalogue record for this book is available from the British Library

Library of Congress Cataloging-in-Publication Data
Carlisle, Susan, 1958-
    Essential clinical skills / Susan Carlisle.
        p. ; cm. -- (Nursing & health survival guides)
    Includes bibliographical references.
    ISBN 978-0-273-76881-4 (pbk.)
    I. Title. II. Series: Nursing & health survival guides.
    [DNLM: 1. Nursing Care--methods--Handbooks. WY 49]

    610.73--dc23

                                            2012002322

10 9 8 7 6 5 4 3 2 1
16 15 14 13 12

Typeset in 8/9.5pt Helvetica by 35
Printed and bound in China (EPC/01)

contents

The Nursing & Midwifery Council states that registered nurses must have the knowledge and skills necessary for safe and effective practice when working. 'Competence is a holistic concept. It is a combination of the skills, knowledge, attitudes, values and technical abilities that underpin safe, effective and autonomous nursing practice' (NMC 2010).

This guide is intended to be a reference tool that will assist nursing students in the safe, competent performance of essential caring activities whilst on their first clinical placements, and assist their mentors in ensuring continuity in the performance of the skills. In addition it is hoped that it will provide guidance to all those healthcare workers who are providing this essential care to patients and clients.

Remember: When performing any procedure, always refer to the practice of your local area (hospital/community).

References

Harver, S., Kozier, B. and Morgan-Samuel, H. (eds) (2011), *Fundamentals of Nursing 2e MyNursingLab Value pack (2nd edition)*, Pearson Education: London

Nursing & Midwifery Council (2010), *Standards for Pre-registration Nurse Education*, NMC London

UK Resuscitation Council (2010), *Adult Basic Life Support Guidelines*, UK Resuscitation Council

introduction

Communication

■ INTERACTING WITH PATIENTS AND CLIENTS

The initial consultation with a patient or client is vital in developing an effective relationship.

INTERACTION	VERBAL SKILL EXAMPLES
Identification	Hello, Mr/Mrs (surname) my name is nursing student (name). It's nice to meet you. How are you?
Introduction	It's a lovely day today, isn't it? Did anyone come with you for your admission today?
Clarification	I would like to ask you some questions to gather some information related to your admission. This will take about 30 minutes.
Consent	Does it suit if I ask you those questions now?
Privacy	Do you mind if I pull the curtains around for some privacy when I am asking you the questions? Does it suit if we go to another room for some privacy when I am asking you the questions?

Examples of non-verbal skills
- Demonstrate a caring approach with warmth/respect/concern.
- Offer a smile/handshake/eye contact/open posture.
- Sit at a similar level to patient/appropriate proximity/head nodding.

- Use appropriate facial expression.
- Maintain an appropriate tone of voice.
- Employ active listening.

All these actions should continue throughout the interaction.

■ THE 'HANDOVER'

In addition to the written record of care, the report or 'handover' plays a significant role in the communication between members of staff and the continuation of patient care. The care plan should be referred to during the handover to ensure that nursing care needs are the main focus when delivering care to patients. The nursing care provided should be evaluated and recorded in a concise and precise manner.

■ NURSING DOCUMENTATION

- Records should be written legibly in black ink in such a way that they cannot be erased and are readable when photocopied.
- Entries must be factual, consistent and accurate and not contain jargon, abbreviations or meaningless phrases.
- Each entry must include the date and time (24-hour clock).
- Each entry must be followed by a signature, the name printed and the job role.
- If an error is made this should be scored out with a single line and the correction written alongside with the date, time and initials of the nurse.
- All entries by nursing students should be countersigned by a registered nurse.

Reference / NMC (2010) *Guidelines for Records and Record Keeping*, Nursing & Midwifery Council, London

Infection control

■ HAND WASHING

Hand washing is important in every setting. It is considered one of the most effective infection control measures.

Hand washing technique

- Turn on the water and adjust the temperature.
- Wet your hands before applying a hand-washing agent.
- Rub your palms together to create a lather.
- Rub the right hand over the back of the left hand with fingers interlaced, change hands and continue.
- Rub your palms together again with fingers interlaced.
- Clasp your fingers together and rub into the palms; change hands and repeat.
- Rotate your right hand around your left thumb.
- Rotate your left hand around your right thumb.
- Use your fingertips to cleanse the centre of your palms.
- Rotate your right hand around your left wrist.
- Rotate your left hand around your right wrist.
- Rinse your hands, shaking off any excess water.
- Dry your hands thoroughly.
- Turn off the taps using your elbows or paper towels.
- Dispose of the paper towels in the household waste bag using the foot pedal.

Figure 1 Eight-step hand hygiene technique

Decontaminate hands using soap and water using the following eight steps. Each step consists of five strokes rubbing backwards and forwards.

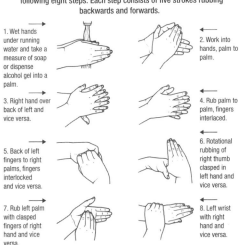

1. Wet hands under running water and take a measure of soap or dispense alcohol gel into a palm.

2. Work into hands, palm to palm.

3. Right hand over back of left and vice versa.

4. Rub palm to palm, fingers interlaced.

5. Back of left fingers to right palms, fingers interlocked and vice versa.

6. Rotational rubbing of right thumb clasped in left hand and vice versa.

7. Rub left palm with clasped fingers of right hand and vice versa.

8. Left wrist with right hand and vice versa.

When using soap and water ensure hands are thoroughly dry before continuing any task

Hands should be washed

- Before and after patient contact.
- After coming in contact with blood or other body fluids.
- After removing protective gloves.
- After using the toilet.
- On leaving the ward.

- Before handling food.
- Between clean and dirty tasks with the same patient.
- Before and after invasive procedures/aseptic techniques.

■ PROTECTIVE CLOTHING

Purpose: to protect healthcare workers and patients from transmission of potentially infective materials.

Disposable gloves should be used if you suspect you will come in contact with blood, body fluids or open wounds.

Disposable aprons should be worn when in direct contact with a patient with a known infection or when contact with blood or other body fluids is likely.

When you have finished the procedure, always dispose of gloves and aprons in the yellow clinical waste bag, making sure you open it using the foot pedal.

■ BED MAKING

When individuals are confined to bed, often for long periods, the bed becomes an important element in their life. A place that is clean, safe and comfortable contributes to the individual's ability to rest and sleep and to a sense of well-being. Making the bed and changing the sheets is an activity which should be performed regularly to ensure a clean, neat environment for the patient and the provision of a smooth, wrinkle-free bed to minimise sources of skin irritation. Care should be taken to prevent spread of infection.

Technique
- Wash your hands and put on disposable apron.
- Ensure the bed is flat and adjusted to a safe, suitable working height.

- Apply the brake on the bed.
- Place new linen on the linen holder.
- Remove used sheets, fold or bunch them neatly.
- Hold used linen away from your own clothes and place them in the laundry bag.
- Put on bottom sheet with sufficient to tuck under mattress.
- Envelope bottom corner at both sides.
- Envelope top corner and tuck in sheet at both sides.
- Ensure sheet is wrinkle-free.
- Complete the bed.
- Readjust the bed height for safety.
- Wash your hands.

■ APPLICATION OF STERILE GLOVES

Purpose: to enable the nurse to handle or touch sterile objects freely without contaminating them and to prevent transmission of potentially infective organisms from the nurse's hands to patients at high risk of infection.

Technique for application
- Wash your hands.
- Clean trolley.
- Check pack and open outer package, emptying content onto trolley.
- Wash your hands.
- Open sterile pack without contaminating inside the package.
- Touch inside of cuff on one glove with finger to lift.
- Pull on first glove without contaminating glove.
- Insert first gloved fingers under cuff of second glove.
- Pull on second glove without contaminating either glove.

- Unfold the cuffs of both gloves without contaminating gloved hand.
- Hold hands away from yourself and above waist after gloves are on.

Technique for removal

- Remove one glove then hold it in the other gloved hand.
- Proceed to remove the second glove, being careful to remove it so that it covers the first glove.
- Grip both sides firmly to ensure that any contamination is held inside the gloves.
- Dispose of both gloves (one glove being wrapped inside the other) in a yellow clinical waste bag.
- Wash your hands and dry thoroughly.

Moving and handling

The importance of safe handling cannot be over emphasised. The priority should at all times be the safety of the patient and the handler.

■ RISK ASSESSMENT

- Task
- Load
- Environment
- Individual capacity

Technique for safe handling

- Never manually handle unless you have no other option. Always ask yourself, 'Do I need to handle manually?'

- Carry out a risk assessment and always select the appropriate manoeuvre and handling equipment for the task in hand.
- Prepare the handling area.
- Wear appropriate clothing and footwear.
- Keep your spine in line. Avoid static stooping.
- Bend the knees when transferring – not the back.
- Use a broad base. Position your feet correctly to reduce spinal rotation.
- Identify a team leader prior to the manoeuvre. All instructions and explanations to both the client and any assisting carers should come from this leader.

Figure 2 Safe handling

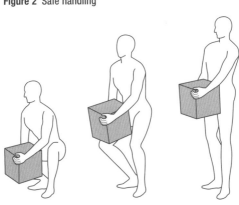

- The leader must give clear, precise instructions (e.g. ready, steady, slide).
- Where appropriate, apply the brakes on equipment. This is so easily forgotten. ***Remember:*** *the exception is the hoist, for which brakes should not be applied unless lifting a client off the floor.*
- Keep the person, or object, to be transferred as close to your body as possible. ***Remember:*** *where necessary, use protective personal equipment.*
- Know your own handling capacity and do not exceed it.
- **If in doubt, seek advice!**

■ POSITIONING OF PATIENTS

The positions used in nursing vary with the needs of the patient. The best position is, if possible, the one the patient finds most comfortable.

POSITION	DESCRIPTION	USES
Recumbent	The patient lies flat on their back with one pillow under the head, arms by the side of their body	• To examine the trunk • To nurse a patient on complete bed rest
Semi-recumbent	The patient lies on their back, half propped up and well supported	• Widely used in medical and surgical nursing • For convalescent patients where no specific position is required

POSITION	DESCRIPTION	USES
Prone	The patient lies flat on their front with the head to one side resting on a pillow. A small pillow is placed under the ankles to prevent the toes pressing on the bed. A second pillow may be placed under the chest	• To relieve pressure • Following back surgery • For patients with extensive back injuries
Semi-prone	The patient lies on one side, but more towards the prone position	• The unconscious patient
Left lateral	The patient lies on the left side, buttocks towards the edge of the bed with the head forward, resting on one pillow, and the thighs and knees bent	• For administering enema and suppositories • Rectal, vaginal and perineal examinations
Dorsal	The patient lies on their back, one pillow under their head, thighs are flexed and knees abducted	• Catheterisation • Abdominal and vaginal examinations

continued

POSITION	DESCRIPTION	USES
Upright	Patient sits straight up in bed or chair. A bed table with a pillow on it may be used to assist the comfort of a breathless patient	• Patients with chronic cardiac and respiratory conditions

Assisting the patient

■ MOBILISING

Patients who have been immobilised for even a few days may require assistance with ambulation (walking). The amount of assistance needed will depend on the individual's condition.

Technique

- Introduce yourself and provide explanation as to the purpose of your intention.
- Select the appropriate walking aid, if necessary.
- Stand next to and slightly behind the patient.
- If the patient requires support, place your arm nearest the patient lightly around their pelvis.
- Your hand should hold the patient's hand closest to you.
- Observe changes in pain as the patient walks.
- Give verbal supervision/cueing as required to achieve safe walking.
- Wash your hands.

■ EATING AND DRINKING

When assisting a patient who has difficulties with eating and drinking, it is important to be sensitive to the patient's feelings. Whenever possible, the carer should help those who may have difficulties to feed themselves.

Technique

- Introduce yourself and give an explanation of what you need to do to gain consent and cooperation.
- Wash your hands thoroughly and wear appropriate protective clothing.
- Ensure the patient is comfortable, i.e. has an empty bladder, clean hands and clean mouth. Help the patient into a comfortable position.
- Allow patient to make their own meal selection.
- Collect and prepare correct food, drink and cutlery and ensure meal is nicely presented.
- Protect the patient's clothing with a napkin.
- Sit down with the patient and ensure the patient is not hurried.
- Tailor the size of each mouthful to the individual patient.
- Assist the patient to take appropriate portions of food at the correct temperature.
- Allow the patient to chew and swallow the food before giving the next mouthful.
- Keep food at a suitable temperature.
- Observe for signs of distress and discontinue as appropriate.
  Remember: take care when placing implements in the patient's mouth.
- Avoid asking questions when the patient is eating, but check between mouthfuls that the food is suitable and the patient is able to continue with the meal.

- Encourage the patient to take as much food as they feel able but do not press if they have indicated they have had sufficient.
- After the meal assist the patient with hygiene needs; for example, wash hands, face and provide mouth care, cleaning teeth. Use the napkin to remove any food particles from the patient's face.
- Ensure patient is comfortable.
- Wash your hands.
- Document and report.

■ TOILETING (BEDPAN/COMMODE USE)

Elimination is a sensitive issue and providing effective care is essential. Potential difficulties can be minimised when the carer seeks to respect the patient's dignity at all times.

Bedpan use

- Explain the procedure to the patient.
- Ensure an appropriate manual handling assessment and action plan is determined.
- Close the door/curtains to ensure privacy.
- Remove the bedclothes to ensure dignity is maintained.
- Put on disposable apron and gloves.
- Assist the patient into the sitting position, unless contraindicated.
- Ask the patient to raise their hips/buttocks then insert the bedpan beneath the patient's pelvis, ensuring the wide end of the bedpan is between the legs and the narrow beneath the buttocks.
- Maintain dignity by ensuring the patient's legs are covered.

- Provide toilet paper and call bell and leave the patient, if their condition allows, but remain nearby.
- When the patient has finished, remove the bedpan and cover and assist the patient with cleaning the perineal area as appropriate.
- Allow the patient the opportunity to wash their hands.
- Ensure the bedclothes are clean, straighten sheets and rearrange pillows.
- Assist the patient into a comfortable position. Ensure the call bell is within easy reach.
- Dispose of the bedpan contents safely after measuring/noting characteristics as appropriate.
- Remove and dispose of apron and gloves.
- Wash your hands.
- Record as appropriate.

Commode use
- Explain the procedure to the patient.
- Ensure an appropriate manual handling assessment and appropriate action plan is determined.
- Put on disposable apron and gloves.
  Take the equipment to the bedside.
- Close the door/curtains to ensure privacy.
- Remove the commode cover and assist the patient out of the bed/chair and onto the commode.
- Once the patient is on the commode, ensure their position is correct.
- Cover the knees with a towel or sheet to maintain privacy and dignity.
- Ensure that toilet paper and call bell are within the patient's reach and, if appropriate, leave the patient but remain nearby.

- When the patient has finished, assist with cleaning the perineal area if necessary.
- Offer the patient the opportunity to wash their hands.
- Assist the patient to bed/chair. Ensure the call bell is within easy reach.
- Replace the cover on the commode and return it to the sluice room.
- Remove the bedpan from underneath the commode and, where necessary, measure the output and note characteristics of contents.
- Dispose of contents safely.
- Clean the commode using warm, soapy water.
- Remove and dispose of apron and gloves.
- Wash your hands.
- Record and report as appropriate.

■ PERSONAL CLEANSING AND DRESSING (BED BATH)

Good personal hygiene is imperative for health and well-being. Patients may require assistance with maintaining their personal hygiene daily. This may be because of a degree of immobility or ill health. Assisting the patient with hygiene needs also gives the carer an opportunity to carry out a comprehensive assessment.

Technique
- Gather equipment required.
- Introduce yourself and explain the procedure to gain the consent and cooperation of the patient.
- Ensure privacy and preserve dignity.
- Wash your hands and put on a plastic apron (gloves are only required if dealing with body fluids or the patient has an infectious disease).

- Ensure water is at the correct temperature.
- With consent, remove top clothes, ensuring the patient is not exposed unnecessarily and is covered with a blanket.
- With consent, remove nightdress/pyjama top. If the patient has a weak arm, take care to remove it from the clothing last to avoid tissue/joint damage.
- Can the patient wash and dry his or her own face? If not, assist them to do this.
- Ensuring dignity and privacy, wash arm farthest away from hand to axilla. Rinse off the soap, dry thoroughly. Repeat with nearest arm.
- With care and sensitivity, uncover chest and abdomen, wash and dry paying particular attention to: skin folds; breasts; dressings in situ; patient's body temperature; how the patient is responding.
- Cover the chest and abdomen; once the patient feels dry apply deodorant, etc., according to the patient's wishes.
- Change water as necessary.
- Sensitively remove lower body clothing.
- Cover nearest leg and place towel under leg furthest away. Wash from toes to groin, rinse and dry thoroughly. Cover leg and repeat with other leg.
- Observe skin, circulation, etc.
- Using a disposable cloth, sensitively wash and dry the genitals and perineal area, working from front to back to minimise risk of contamination of urethra/vagina with faecal matter.
- Change water, use a clean cloth and ask the patient to roll over or seek help to roll the patient onto their side.
- Wash and dry back and buttocks, in particular observing the skin along pressure points.
- Change sheets and assist with dressing the patient in fresh nightclothes.

- Attend to oral hygiene, hair care, spectacles and any other personal requirements.
- Remove apron and wash your hands.

Observation of vital signs

■ TEMPERATURE

Measurement of body temperature is carried out:

1. To determine a baseline
2. To monitor fluctuations in temperature

> **Key fact:** Body temperature is usually maintained between 36°C and 37.5°C.

Digital thermometer technique

- Introduce yourself and explain to the patient the purpose of recording temperature in order to gain consent and cooperation.
- Ensure patient is in a comfortable position.
- Collect equipment and wash your hands.
- Remove protective cap from thermometer and check the symbol on the display.
- Apply new probe cover.
- Lift the pinna of the ear (flap of skin and cartilage that projects from the head) and gently insert the probe into the auditory canal.
- Keep the thermometer in position until an audible tone signals the correct temperature has been reached.
- Read the display.
- Discard the probe cover into a yellow clinical waste bag.
- Replace the protective cap on the probe.

- Wash your hands.
- Record/report the temperature.

Single-use clinical thermometer technique
Oral use:
- Place under the tongue as far back as possible.
- Have the patient press the tongue down on the thermometer and keep the mouth closed for 60 seconds.
- Remove the thermometer. Some blue dots may disappear as the device locks in for accuracy.
- Read the last blue dot; ignore any skipped dot.
- Discard thermometer.
- Wash your hands.
- Record temperature.

Axillary use:
- Position thermometer high in the armpit, vertical to the body, with the dots against the torso.
- Lower the patient's arm to hold the thermometer in place.
- Remove the thermometer after 3 minutes.
- Discard thermometer.
- Wash your hands.
- Record temperature.

■ PULSE

Pulse is taken to gather information on the heart rate, rhythm (pattern of beats) and strength of pulse. Measurement is carried out:
1. To determine the individual's pulse as a baseline
2. To monitor changes

Key fact: The normal pulse rate per minute for an adult ranges from 55 to 90 beats per minute.

Figure 3 Locations of pulse in the body

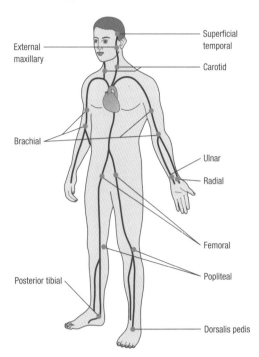

Technique

- Introduce yourself and explain to the patient the purpose of measuring and recording the pulse in order to gain consent and cooperation.
- Ensure the patient's arm is in a comfortable resting position.
- Locate the radial artery at the base of the thumb.
- Place the first, second or third fingers of the dominant hand along the artery and press gently.
- Count the number of beats for 60 seconds. Note: rate, rhythm, character, volume.
- Wash your hands.
- Record pulse and report any abnormality.

■ RESPIRATION

Respiration is measured:
1. To determine a baseline respiratory rate
2. To monitor changes in respiration
3. To evaluate the patient's response to medications or treatments that affect the respiratory system

> **Key fact:** The average rate for an adult is 15–20 breaths per minute.

Technique

- Continue to hold the patient's wrist for a further 60 seconds while counting the respirations.
- Count every rise and fall of the chest as one respiration.

- Leave the patient comfortable.
- Wash your hands.
- Record/report the respiration rate, reporting any abnormality. Note the rhythm or depth as appropriate.

■ BLOOD PRESSURE

Blood pressure is monitored:
1. To determine a baseline
2. To monitor fluctuations

> **Key fact:** Blood pressure in an adult generally ranges from 100/60 to 140/90 mmHg. However, this can fluctuate within a wide range and still be considered normal.

Manual blood pressure technique
- Introduce yourself and explain the procedure in order to gain the consent and cooperation of the patient.
- Wash your hands.
- Ensure the patient has been resting for 5 minutes and has not eaten for 30 minutes.
- Assist the patient into a comfortable position; ensure the arm is at heart level, resting on a suitable firm surface.
- Ensure the arm is free from restrictive clothing.

Figure 4 Steps to taking accurate measurements

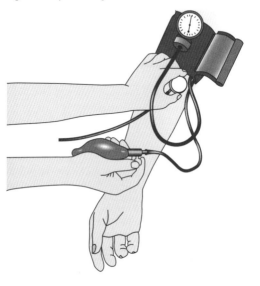

- Palpate the brachial/radial artery.
- Apply the cuff around the arm smoothly and firmly with the bladder centred over the brachial artery 2.5 centimetres above the ante-cubital fossa (the depression at the front of the elbow).
- Position the sphygmomanometer at heart level, ensuring that the mercury level is at zero and can be easily read.
- Connect the cuff tubing and close the valve to create a sealed unit within the equipment.
- Remind the patient of the feeling of tightness in the arm as the cuff is inflated, emphasising that this is temporary.
- Palpate the radial artery and inflate the cuff until the pulse is no longer palpable (this will give an approximate value of the systolic pressure). Deflate the cuff rapidly, wait 15–30 seconds, then check the mercury level is at zero.
- Clean the earpieces of the stethoscope.
- Position the stethoscope over the brachial artery and inflate the cuff 2–3 mmHg per second to 30 mmHg above the previously determined pressure.
- Deflate the cuff at a rate of 2–3 mmHg per second and note when the first two consecutive beats are heard. This is the systolic pressure.
- Continue to deflate the cuff and note when the beats disappear. This is the diastolic pressure (listen for 10–20 mmHg below the disappearance of the sound).
- Completely deflate the cuff, disconnect the tubing and remove the cuff from the patient's arm.
- Clean the earpieces of the stethoscope.
- Leave the patient comfortable.

- Wash your hands.
- Record and report the measurement accurately to the nearest 2 mmHg.

■ WEIGHING THE PATIENT

Data including weight can be vital in evaluating the nutritional status of a patient.

Technique
- Introduce yourself and explain the purpose of the procedure in order to gain consent.
- Position the scales for easy access and apply the brakes (if appropriate).
- Ask the patient to remove shoes and outdoor garments. The patient should be wearing light indoor clothes only.
- Ensure that the scales are at zero then ask the patient to stand/sit on these.
- Ask the patient to remain still.
- Note the reading on the scale and record immediately, taking care that it is legible.

Eye care

Eye care is performed to maintain healthy eyes through keeping them moist and infection-free.

Technique
- Introduce yourself and explain the procedure in order to gain consent.
- Clean the trolley and collect the equipment you require.

- Assist the patient into the correct position (either lying or seated with head tilted back).
- Ensure you have adequate light.
- Wash hands and apply gloves.
- Using a slightly moistened swab, ask the patient to look up and swab the lower eyelid from the lower corner outwards.
- Using a new swab each time, repeat until the discharge is removed.
- Repeat the procedure for the upper lid, asking the patient to look down.
- Dry the lids with a dry swab.
- Assess the patient's comfort.
- Remove and dispose of the equipment in a clinical waste bag.
- Wash your hands and dry thoroughly.
- Record and report accordingly.

Mouth care

Good oral hygiene is essential. Certain patients are prone to oral problems because of lack of knowledge or the inability to maintain oral hygiene.

Technique
- Introduce yourself and explain the procedure in order to gain consent and cooperation.
- Collect necessary equipment.
- Wash your hands and put on an apron and gloves.
- Place tissues under the patient's chin.
- Ask the patient to open their mouth wide.

- Inspect the patient's mouth, especially the buccal mucosa, with the aid of a torch and spatula.
- Using a toothbrush and toothpaste/teledont, brush the patient's teeth and gums.
- Keep the brush positioned over only two or three teeth at a time. Use small rotating movements to cover the outside surfaces of all teeth.
- Clean the inner surfaces of all back teeth and the buccal cavity the same way.
- Examine the condition of the teeth and gums and mucus membranes.
- If the patient is unable to rinse, use a rinsed toothbrush to clean the teeth and moistened foam sticks to wipe gums and oral mucosa.
- Lubricate the patient's lips with petroleum jelly.
- Remove gloves and apron and dispose of all equipment correctly.
- Wash hands.
- Record and report accordingly.

Wound care (simple dressing)

The aim of wound cleaning is to create an optimum environment for healing by the removal of excess debris, exudate, bacteria and other micro-organisms.

Technique

- Introduce yourself and explain the procedure to gain the patient's consent.
- Clean the dressing trolley and assemble sufficient quantity of required equipment.

- Position the patient comfortably to allow access to the wound site.
- Wash your hands and put on an apron.
- Check the pack and open it using the non-touch technique.
- Wash your hands and arrange the contents of the pack using the waste bag.
- Remove the soiled dressing using the waste bag and invert.
- Hang the bag on the side of the trolley.
- Open any accessory material as required.
- Wash your hands.
- Put on sterile gloves.
- Using your gloved hand, irrigate the wound and dry the surrounding area with a fresh swab.
- Apply suitable dressing with gloved hand.
- Make the patient comfortable.
- Discard disposable items and place soiled dressings, etc. in the clinical waste bag.
- Wash hands.
- Record and report.

Catheter care

Cleaning the urethral meatus (where the catheter enters the body) is a procedure intended to minimise infection.

Technique
- Introduce yourself to the patient and explain the procedure in order to allay anxiety and gain consent.
- Collect and prepare equipment.
- Assist the patient into a suitable position, maintaining dignity.

- Wash your hands.
- Put on an apron and gloves.
- Gently cleanse the external urethral meatus (opening) using the wipe only once and in one direction, wiping from above downwards and away from the catheter-meatal junction.
- Gently wipe the shaft of the catheter away from the catheter-meatal junction.
- Ensure that the area is dry using clean dry wipes.
- Ensure you show concern for the patient's feelings and dignity throughout.
- Dispose of the equipment safely and appropriately.
- Remove and dispose of gloves.
- Wash your hands.
- Record and report appropriately.

■ EMPTYING A URINARY CATHETER BAG

Technique

- Introduce yourself and explain the procedure in order to gain the consent and cooperation of the patient.
- Wash your hands thoroughly and put on disposable gloves.
- Clean the outlet valve with an alcohol-saturated swab.
- Allow the urine to drain into a jug.
- Close the outlet valve and clean it again with a new alcohol-saturated swab.
- Cover the jug and, if required, note the amount of urine for fluid balance records. Dispose of the contents in the sluice.
- Remove and dispose of gloves. Wash your hands thoroughly.

Specimen collection

A general assessment of the patient involves a number of tasks, including the collection of different specimens.

Technique
- Introduce yourself and explain the purpose of the procedure in order to gain consent and cooperation.
- Wash your hands thoroughly and wear appropriate protective clothing.
- Ensure privacy and maintain patient's dignity whilst specimen is being collected/provided.
- Place the specimen in the appropriate, correctly labelled container.
- Wash your hands.
- Dispatch the specimen to the laboratory promptly with the completed request form.

Urinalysis

Urinalysis is an important diagnostic test used to assess for conditions such as urinary tract infections and renal calculi. The urine can be tested using reagent strips, and if used according to the manufacturer's guidelines are relatively accurate.

Technique
- Wash your hands.
- Collect urinalysis test strips.
- Put on gloves and apron.
- Observe the colour of the urine.

- Observe if there is sediment present.
- Observe and note the odour of the urine.
- Check the expiry date of the reagent strips.
- Remove a reagent strip without touching the test square on the strip.
- Recap the container.
- Dip the reagent strip fully into the urine and accurately note the time.
- Tap the reagent strip against the top of the container to remove any excess urine.
- Wait the recommended time, keeping the strip horizontal and ensuring it does not touch the container.
- Read the strip, comparing the colour on the reagent strip to the colour code on the container at the appropriate times.
- Discard the reagent strip into the yellow clinical waste disposal bag using the foot pedal.
- Remove and dispose of gloves and apron.
- Wash your hands.
- Record the result and report any abnormality.

Peak flow

Peak flow is a measurement of the highest rate at which air can be expelled from the lungs through an open mouth. It is a useful aid in diagnosing and monitoring asthma and respiratory conditions.

Technique

- Introduce yourself and explain the purpose of peak flow in order to gain the patient's consent and cooperation.

- Wash your hands.
- Ensure the patient is in the correct position, standing if possible or sitting fully upright.
- Fit a clean disposable mouthpiece to the peak flow meter and ensure that the flow indicator is at zero.
- Instruct the patient to take a deep breath, clamp lips around the mouthpiece and blow out as hard as possible in a short, sharp manner.
- Note the number on the scale indicated by the pointer, return the pointer to zero.
- Repeat the procedure twice more to obtain three readings.
- Monitor the patient for fatigue and technique. Encourage patient effort.
- Leave the patient comfortable.
- Dispose of the mouthpiece in the yellow clinical waste bag.
- Wash your hands.
- Report and record accurately the best of the three readings.

Oxygen administration

Patients who have difficulty ventilating all areas of their lungs, those whose gas exchange is impaired, or people with heart failure, may require oxygen therapy to prevent hypoxia. Oxygen therapy is a prescribed medication.

Technique
- Introduce yourself and explain to the patient the purpose of oxygen therapy in order to gain consent and cooperation.

- Wash your hands.
- Check the prescription on the medicine kardex to identify the percentage of oxygen to be administered.
- Collect the appropriate mask and valve and attach the tubing to the mask and oxygen supply.
- Check the patient's identification with the prescription sheet prior to commencement of the therapy.
- Assist the patient into an upright position ensuring comfort.
- Explain the dangers of smoking; ensure a no smoking sign is placed above the patient's bed – this is particularly important if the patient is at home or not in a hospital with a no-smoking policy.
- Turn on the oxygen, ensure there is no leakage.
- Set the flow rate according to the prescription to ensure the correct percentage of oxygen is administered.
- Check the oxygen is flowing by listening or feeling. Allow the patient to feel the oxygen against their cheek or hand prior to administration via the facemask.
- When the patient is ready, secure the mask ensuring it is comfortable.
- Stay with the patient for a few moments to ensure compliance.
- Leave the patient comfortable.
- Wash your hands.
- Record that oxygen therapy has commenced, stating the percentage and rate of flow and noting patient compliance. Report accordingly.

Medicine administration

The Nursing & Midwifery Council (2008) Standards for Medicines Management establish the standards that all registered nurses are expected to work to when administering drugs.

When administering medication the prescription should

- Be based on the patient's informed consent and awareness of the purpose of the treatment.
- Be clearly written and indelible.
- Clearly identify the patient for whom the medication is intended.
- Record the weight of the patient where the dose is related to weight.
- Clearly specify the substance to be administered, its generic name, its stated form, the strength, dosage, timing and frequency of administration, start and finish dates and route of administration.
- Be signed and dated by the authorised prescriber.
- Not be for a substance to which the patient is allergic or unable to tolerate.
- In the case of controlled drugs, specify the dosage and number of dosage units or total course.

You must

- Know the therapeutic uses of the medicine, its dosage, side effects, precautions and contra-indications.
- Be certain of the identity of the patient.
- Be aware of the patient's care plan.

- Check the prescription and the label on the medicine is clearly written and unambiguous.
- Have considered the dosage, method, route and timing in the context of the condition of the patient and co-existing therapies.
- Check the patient is not allergic to the medicine.
- Contact the prescriber without delay where contra-indications to the prescribed medication are discovered, where a patient develops a reaction to the medicine or where assessment of the patient indicates that the medicine is no longer suitable.
- Make a clear, accurate and immediate record of all medicine administered, intentionally withheld or refused by the patient, ensuring that written entries and the signature are clear and legible.
- Make sure that a record is made when delegating the task of administering medicine.
- The supervising registered nurse should countersign student's signatures.

Drug calculation:

$$\frac{\text{Prescribed dose} \times \text{Vol}}{\text{Stock dose}} = \text{Amount to be administered}$$

Action in the event of a needlestick injury

Remember: Always maintain sharps awareness.
Dispose of needles and other sharps safely.

- Encourage bleeding from the affected site.
- Wash the injured area/irrigate.

- Cover with a waterproof dressing.
- Report to line manager.
- Attempt to identify source patient and assess risk.
- Complete an accident/incident form.
- Seek medical help as soon as possible – go to Occupational health or A&E or your GP.

Basic life support

■ SEQUENCE OF ACTION

1. Check safety.
2. Check response.
3. If no response shout for help.
4. Open airway with head tilt/chin lift and check for breathing (up to 10 seconds).

Unconscious casualty (breathing)

- Put in recovery position.
- Check for continued breathing.
- Get help.

Unconscious casualty (not breathing)

- Send (or go) for help. Dial 999 (Automated External Defibrillates; AED).
- Commence chest compressions.
- Combine chest compressions and rescue breathing at a ratio of 30:2.
- Continue resuscitation until
  - the victim shows signs of life,
  - qualified help arrives,
  - you become exhausted.

Figure 5 Adult basic life support

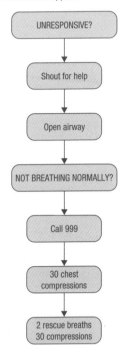

Resuscitation Council (UK)

■ CPR TECHNIQUE

- Place the heel of one hand in the centre of the chest and place the heel of the other hand on top of the first hand.
- Interlock the fingers of your hands and ensure that pressure is not applied over the ribs.
- Do not apply pressure over the upper abdomen or the bottom end of the sternum.
- Position yourself vertically above the chest and, keeping arms straight, press down on the sternum, depressing it by 5–6 centimetres.
- After each compression release all the pressure on the chest without losing contact between the hands and sternum.
- Use a compression rate of 100–120 per minute.
- After 30 compressions, establish airway.
- Give two rescue breaths, checking for rise and fall of chest.
- Continue at a ratio of 30:2.

■ RECOVERY POSITION

On finding the collapsed casualty:

1. Check safety.
2. Check response.
3. If no response, shout for help.
4. Open airway with head tilt/chin lift and check for breathing (up to 10 seconds).

Following assessment, if you find the unconscious casualty is breathing, place in the recovery position and seek appropriate help.

Figure 6 Recovery position

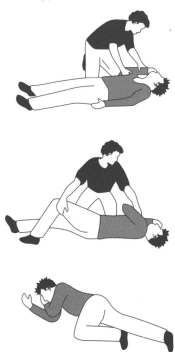

Technique

- Remove the casualty's glasses, if present.
- Kneel beside the casualty and make sure that both legs are straight.
- Place the arm nearest to you out at right angles to their body, elbow bent with the hand palm-up.
- Bring the far arm across the chest and hold the back of the hand against the casualty's cheek nearest to you.
- With your other hand, grasp the far leg just above the knee and pull it up, keeping the foot on the ground.
- Keeping the casualty's hand pressed against their cheek, pull on the far leg to roll them towards you onto their side.
- Adjust the upper leg so that both the hip and knee are bent at right angles.
- Tilt the head back to make sure that the airway remains open.
- If necessary, adjust the hand under the cheek to keep the head tilted and facing downwards to allow liquid material to drain from the mouth.
- Check breathing regularly.
- If the casualty has to be kept in the recovery position for more than half an hour, turn them onto their other side after 30 minutes.

■ ADULT CHOKING TREATMENT (this is appropriate for a child over 1 year)

Figure 7 Adult choking treatment algorithm

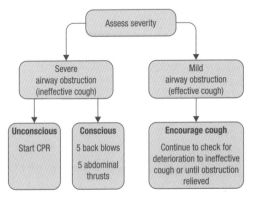

Resuscitation Council (UK)

If the casualty shows signs of mild obstruction
• Encourage coughing

If the casualty shows signs of severe obstruction
• Support the casualty and give up to five back blows between the shoulders with the heel of your hand.
• If this fails to relieve the obstruction, give up to five abdominal thrusts.
• Continue alternating five back blows with five abdominal thrusts until the obstruction is relieved.